GAO

United States Government Accountability Office

Report to Congressional Requesters

December 2011

MEDICARE ADVANTAGE

Changes Improved Accuracy of Risk Adjustment for Certain Beneficiaries

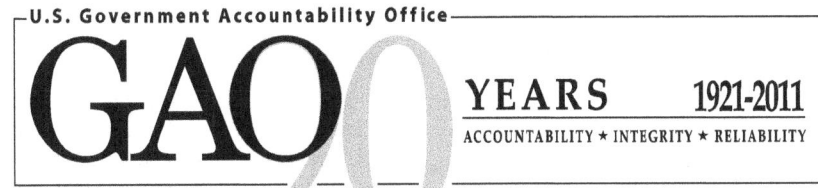

GAO-12-52

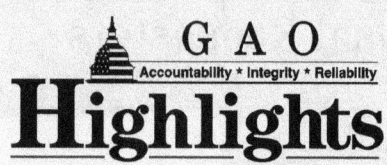

December 2011

MEDICARE ADVANTAGE
Changes Improved Accuracy of Risk Adjustment for Certain Beneficiaries

Highlights of GAO-12-52, a report to congressional requesters

Why GAO Did This Study

The Centers for Medicare & Medicaid Services (CMS) pays plans in Medicare Advantage (MA)—the private plan alternative to Medicare fee-for-service (FFS)—an amount per beneficiary that is adjusted to reflect beneficiary health status. This adjustment, called risk adjustment, helps ensure that health plans have the same financial incentive to enroll and care for beneficiaries regardless of their health status. In 2010, CMS announced plans to revise the major medical conditions included in its principal risk-adjustment model—the community model—and add a model for new enrollees in chronic condition special needs plans (C-SNP), which target beneficiaries with certain severe or disabling chronic conditions. CMS began using the C-SNP new enrollee model in 2011, in place of the general new enrollee model, to adjust MA payments for new Medicare beneficiaries who enroll in a C-SNP. GAO was asked to examine the accuracy of these models for high-risk beneficiaries. Using data for a nationally representative sample of 2007 FFS beneficiaries, GAO computed the amount that expenditure estimates were above or below actual expenditures for 2007, the most recent data available at the time. GAO compared the accuracy of the current and revised community models for three high-risk groups: beneficiaries with multiple chronic conditions, with low income, and with dementia. GAO compared the accuracy of the general and C-SNP new enrollee models for new enrollees eligible to enroll in a C-SNP.

View GAO-12-52. For more information, contact James C. Cosgrove at (202) 512-7114 or cosgrovej@gao.gov.

What GAO Found

The effect of CMS's revised community model on payment accuracy varied for the high-risk groups studied. Specifically, compared with the current community model, the revised community model slightly reduced the accuracy of MA payment adjustments for beneficiaries with multiple chronic conditions by $164, or about 1 percent of average actual expenditures. For beneficiaries with low income, the accuracy of the revised and the current community models was similar: estimates differed by $5, or less than 0.1 percent of average actual expenditures. For beneficiaries with dementia, the revised community model substantially improved the accuracy of MA payment adjustments by $2,674, or about 16 percent of average actual expenditures.

Compared with the general new enrollee model, the C-SNP new enrollee model substantially improved the accuracy of MA payment adjustments for new enrollees with C-SNP conditions, but considerable inaccuracy in the model's estimates remains for certain groups. The amount by which accuracy improved was similar across 14 severe or disabling chronic conditions: about $2,500. This reflects the design of the C-SNP new enrollee model, which increases expenditure estimates from the general new enrollee model by an amount that does not depend on beneficiaries' medical conditions. However, the C-SNP new enrollee model still underestimated expenditures for C-SNP-eligible new enrollees, on average, by about $1,500 and by more than $15,000 for beneficiaries who had certain conditions, such as end-stage liver disease or stroke. The C-SNP new enrollee model's results varied depending on the number of severe or disabling conditions the beneficiary had. Specifically, the model reduced the accuracy of estimated expenditures for new enrollees with only 1 severe or disabling condition by about 62 percent of average actual expenditures but improved the accuracy for those with 4 or more conditions by about 8 percent. However, the C-SNP new enrollee model still underestimated expenditures for beneficiaries with 4 or more conditions by over $20,000.

Accurate risk adjustment is particularly important for certain high-risk beneficiary groups that are more challenging and costly to treat and may benefit particularly from the coordination of care MA plans can provide. The decision to implement the revised community model that adjusts for dementia will depend on CMS's assessment of the advantages of more accurate payment adjustment for beneficiaries with dementia compared with the potential increase in the discretionary coding of dementia because of revised coding guidelines for Alzheimer's disease dementia published in April 2011. Additionally, while the introduction of the C-SNP new enrollee model improved the accuracy of payment adjustments for eligible new enrollees, on average, the model still considerably underestimated expenditures for certain groups, which could place plans that disproportionately enroll beneficiaries in these groups at a relative financial disadvantage.

In its comments on a draft of this report, CMS suggested that GAO assess the overall accuracy of the current risk adjustment model. GAO did not assess overall model accuracy because such an analysis was not within the scope of GAO's work and would have required additional data.

United States Government Accountability Office

Contents

Letter		1
	Background	7
	Effect of Revised Community Model on Payment Accuracy Varied for High-Risk Groups Studied	10
	C-SNP New Enrollee Model Substantially Improved Accuracy of MA Payment Adjustments, but Considerable Inaccuracy Remains for Certain Groups	15
	Concluding Observations	18
	Agency Comments and Our Evaluation	19
Appendix I	Additional Potential Changes to the Medicare Advantage Risk-Adjustment Models	22
Appendix II	Scope and Methodology	26
Appendix III	Comments from the Centers for Medicare & Medicaid Services	31
Appendix IV	GAO Contact and Staff Acknowledgments	34
Tables		
	Table 1: Potential Changes to the Medicare Advantage (MA) Risk-Adjustment Models: Adding Variables to the Models	23
	Table 2: Potential Changes to the Medicare Advantage (MA) Risk-Adjustment Models: Adding New Information Sources	24
	Table 3: Potential Changes to the Medicare Advantage (MA) Risk-Adjustment Models: Changing Models' Structure	25
Figures		
	Figure 1: Accuracy of Current and Revised Community Models' Estimated Health Care Expenditures for Beneficiaries, by Number of Chronic Conditions, 2007	11

Figure 2: Accuracy of Current and Revised Community Models' Estimated Health Care Expenditures for Beneficiaries, by Income Status, 2007   13

Figure 3: Accuracy of Current and Revised Community Models' Estimated Health Care Expenditures for Beneficiaries, by Dementia Diagnosis, 2007   14

Figure 4: Accuracy of General and Chronic Condition Special Needs Plan (C-SNP) New Enrollee Models' Estimated Health Care Expenditures for New Enrollees, by Severe or Disabling Chronic Condition, 2007   16

Figure 5: Accuracy of General and Chronic Condition Special Needs Plan (C-SNP) New Enrollee Models' Estimated Health Care Expenditures for New Enrollees, by Number of Severe or Disabling Chronic Conditions, 2007   18

Abbreviations

ADLs	activities of daily living
C-SNP	chronic condition special needs plan
CMS	Centers for Medicare & Medicaid Services
CMS-HCC	CMS-Hierarchical Condition Category
DME	durable medical equipment
ESRD	end-stage renal disease
FFS	fee-for-service
HCC	hierarchical condition category
LIS	low-income subsidy
MA	Medicare Advantage

This is a work of the U.S. government and is not subject to copyright protection in the United States. The published product may be reproduced and distributed in its entirety without further permission from GAO. However, because this work may contain copyrighted images or other material, permission from the copyright holder may be necessary if you wish to reproduce this material separately.

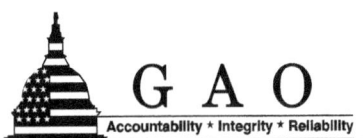

United States Government Accountability Office
Washington, DC 20548

December 9, 2011

Congressional Requesters

In 2010, the federal government spent approximately $114 billion on the Medicare Advantage (MA) program, which covered nearly a quarter of all Medicare beneficiaries. The MA program is an alternative to the original Medicare fee-for-service (FFS) program,[1] in which private health insurance plans offer health care coverage to Medicare beneficiaries. MA plans are required to enroll all eligible Medicare beneficiaries who apply, regardless of their health status.[2] The Centers for Medicare & Medicaid Services (CMS), which administers Medicare, pays MA plans a monthly amount per beneficiary that is adjusted to reflect beneficiary health status—a process known as risk adjustment. Accurate risk adjustment helps ensure that health plans have the same financial incentive to enroll and care for beneficiaries regardless of their health status and avoids the creation of a financial advantage or disadvantage for health plans solely on the basis of the health status of enrolled beneficiaries.

CMS uses risk-adjustment models to adjust payments to MA plans.[3] These models use a beneficiary's characteristics to estimate the amount Medicare FFS would be expected to spend to provide care for that beneficiary. CMS compares this estimate with the actual average expenditure per Medicare FFS beneficiary and adjusts MA payments by that ratio. For example, payments to MA plans are doubled for beneficiaries whose health care expenditures are estimated to be twice as high as the average FFS expenditure. Most payments are risk

---

[1]Medicare FFS consists of Medicare Parts A and B. Medicare Part A provides coverage for hospital and other inpatient stays. Medicare Part B is optional insurance and provides coverage for hospital outpatient, physician, and other services. Medicare beneficiaries have the option of obtaining coverage for Medicare Part A and B services from private health plans that participate in the MA program—also known as Medicare Part C. Medicare beneficiaries may purchase optional coverage for outpatient prescription drugs under Medicare Part D.

[2]Medicare beneficiaries with Part A and Part B who live in the service area of an MA plan and who do not have end-stage renal disease (ESRD) are generally eligible to join an MA plan.

[3]Risk-adjustment models are designed to accurately estimate average health care expenditures for groups of beneficiaries with similar characteristics, but not necessarily to accurately estimate expenditures for each individual in those groups.

adjusted using expenditure estimates from CMS's community model. The community model uses a beneficiary's demographic information and major medical conditions from a base year to estimate health care expenditures during the following year.[4] CMS uses a different model, called the general new enrollee model, for most beneficiaries with less than 1 complete calendar year of Medicare Part B enrollment.[5] This model estimates expenditures solely based on beneficiaries' demographic information.

Some research has shown that CMS's community risk-adjustment model systematically overestimates health care expenditures for some beneficiary groups and underestimates expenditures for others.[6] Of particular interest is the degree of the model's accuracy in estimating health care expenditures for certain high-risk beneficiary groups, which are more challenging and costly to treat and may benefit particularly from the coordination of care MA plans can provide. These groups include beneficiaries with multiple chronic conditions, low income levels, and dementia.[7] For instance, one study found that the community risk-adjustment model underestimated expenditures for beneficiaries with dementia by nearly 16 percent.[8] The potentially inaccurate estimation of

---

[4]There are 70 major medical conditions, called hierarchical condition categories (HCC), included in the current community model. These major medical conditions contain a broad set of similar diagnoses that are related clinically and with respect to costs.

[5]CMS uses a separate new enrollee model for beneficiaries with ESRD who have less than 1 full calendar year of Medicare Part B enrollment.

[6]Some researchers who have compared actual beneficiary expenditures with expenditures estimated from the community risk-adjustment model noted that the community model systematically underpredicts expenditures for beneficiaries with above-average costs and overpredicts expenditures for those with below-average costs. See Jason Brown et al., "How Does Risk Selection Respond to Risk Adjustment? Evidence from the Medicare Advantage Program," National Bureau of Economic Research Working Paper number 16977 (April 2011).

[7]Studies have shown that low-income beneficiaries, such as dual-eligibles (beneficiaries eligible for Medicare and Medicaid), have high expected health care expenditures. For example, see Medicare Payment Advisory Commission, "Coordinating the Care of Dual-Eligible Beneficiaries," in *Report to the Congress: Aligning Incentives in Medicare* (Washington, D.C.: June 2010), and Teresa Coughlin, Timothy Waidmann, and Molly O'Malley Watts, "Where Does the Burden Lie? Medicaid and Medicare Spending for Dual Eligible Beneficiaries" (Kaiser Commission on Medicaid and the Uninsured, April 2009).

[8]See Katia Noyes, Hangshen Lui, and Helena Temkin-Greener, "Medicare Capitation Model, Functional Status, and Multiple Comorbidities: Model Accuracy," *The American Journal of Managed Care*, vol. 14, no. 10, (2008): 679-690.

Medicare expenditures for high-risk beneficiary groups may be especially relevant for new enrollees in chronic condition special needs plans (C-SNP)—plans that only enroll beneficiaries with at least 1 of 15 severe or disabling chronic conditions—because the general new enrollee risk-adjustment model does not account for the severe or disabling condition(s) that an individual must have to enroll in a C-SNP.[9,10] While there are relatively few C-SNP new enrollees—fewer than 10,000 in 2010—accurate risk-adjustment is especially important for this group of beneficiaries as they may benefit particularly from the coordination of care C-SNPs can provide.

CMS has been conducting ongoing research on how to improve the accuracy of its MA risk-adjustment models and, in 2010, announced its plans to implement two major changes.[11] First, CMS proposed revising the major medical conditions included in the community model. CMS initially planned to implement this revised community model in 2011 but has since announced that the model would not be implemented in 2011 or 2012.[12] Second, CMS created a new risk-adjustment model to adjust payments for new enrollees who enrolled in C-SNPs. Like the general

---

[9] The 15 severe and disabling chronic conditions for which C-SNPs can target enrollment are alcohol and other drug dependence, autoimmune disorders, cancer (excluding precancer conditions or in situ status), cardiovascular disorders, chronic heart failure, dementia, diabetes mellitus, end-stage liver disease, ESRD, severe hematological disorders, Human Immunodeficiency Virus/Acquired Immunodeficiency Syndrome, chronic lung disorders, chronic and disabling mental health conditions, neurological disorders, and stroke. The 15 conditions were defined by a panel of clinical advisors convened by CMS.

[10] In addition to C-SNPs, there are two other types of special needs plans—one that enrolls beneficiaries who reside in long-term care facilities and another that enrolls beneficiaries who are dual-eligible.

[11] A summary of additional modifications to the MA community risk-adjustment models that CMS considered but did not propose for implementation is in app. I.

[12] CMS originally postponed implementation of the revised community model from 2011 to 2012 because of statutory provisions enacted in 2010 regarding MA payment methodology. Because multiple MA payment changes are scheduled for implementation in 2012, CMS decided not to adjust MA plan payments using the revised community model in 2012. However, CMS stated that it would use the revised community model to adjust payments to certain non-MA plans, which provide a managed care benefit for individuals who are age 55 or older and require a certain level of nursing care. See CMS, "Announcement of Calendar Year (CY) 2011 Medicare Advantage Capitation Rates and Medicare Advantage and Part D Payment Policies and Final Call Letter" (Apr. 5, 2010), and "Announcement of Calendar Year (CY) 2012 Medicare Advantage Capitation Rates and Medicare Advantage and Part D Payment Policies and Final Call Letter" (Apr. 4, 2011).

new enrollee model, the C-SNP new enrollee model only uses beneficiaries' demographic characteristics to estimate expenditures. However, to account for the relatively higher expected health care expenditures for C-SNP new enrollees compared with the average new enrollee in Medicare, the C-SNP new enrollee model estimates higher expenditures than the general new enrollee model for beneficiaries with the same set of demographic characteristics. CMS began adjusting MA payments using the C-SNP new enrollee model in 2011.

Given the importance of accurate risk adjustment, you asked us to examine how accurately the MA risk-adjustment models estimate health care expenditures, especially for high-risk beneficiary groups. This report compares (1) the accuracy with which the current and revised community models adjust MA payments to account for differences in beneficiaries' expected health care expenditures and (2) the accuracy with which the general and C-SNP new enrollee models adjust MA payments to account for differences in beneficiaries' expected health care expenditures.

To compare the accuracy with which the current and revised community models would adjust MA payments, we computed the amount by which health care expenditure estimates from the current and revised community models were above or below actual expenditures. We calculated the accuracy of the average estimated health expenditures for a particular group of beneficiaries by subtracting the average actual annualized Medicare expenditures in 2007 from the average estimated annual expenditures for 2007. We considered the revised model an improvement in accuracy of MA payment adjustments if the magnitude of the over- or underestimate of health care expenditures from the revised model was smaller than the over- or underestimate from the current model. For example, if the revised model overestimated expenditures by $100 and the current model underestimated expenditures by $200, this indicated that the revised model improved accuracy because the magnitude of the over- or underestimate was smaller than the magnitude for the current model.

For this analysis, we used versions of the current and revised community models that differed only in the diagnoses that were included in the models.[13] We analyzed data on annualized Medicare expenditures and diagnostic and demographic information for a 5 percent nationally representative, random sample of 2007 Medicare FFS community beneficiaries,[14] which was the most recent version of these data available. The beneficiaries in our sample are those who, if they had enrolled in an MA plan, would have had their 2007 payments adjusted by the community model. We used data on beneficiaries in Medicare FFS because health care expenditure data were not available for MA beneficiaries.

Using these data, we compared the accuracy of the current and revised community models for three high-risk beneficiary groups separately. We defined these three groups as follows based on their characteristics in the previous year:[15]

- diagnosed with multiple chronic conditions among those included in the revised community model;

- low income, which we defined as being dually eligible for Medicare and Medicaid or receiving the Part D low-income subsidy (LIS);[16] and

- diagnosed with dementia with or without complications.

---

[13]The revised community model was also recalibrated with more recent data from 2006 and 2007. (The current model was calibrated with data from 2004 and 2005.) However, because CMS performs such updates on a periodic basis, we focused our analysis on the impact of changes in the HCCs included in the model. We did so by comparing the revised community model with a version of the current community model that was also calibrated with data from 2006 and 2007.

[14]Community beneficiaries are those with a complete year of Medicare Part B enrollment during the previous calendar year who have not been diagnosed with ESRD and have not been residing in an institution, such as a nursing home, for at least the previous 90 days. In 2010, more than 90 percent of MA beneficiaries had their payments adjusted with the community model.

[15]Because the community model is a prospective model, expenditure estimates from one year are based on beneficiaries' characteristics in the previous year. For our sample of 2007 Medicare FFS community beneficiaries, we therefore identified our high-risk beneficiary groups based on our sample's characteristics in 2006.

[16]The Part D LIS program provides financial assistance to beneficiaries with limited income and assets. Eligible beneficiaries include those with annual incomes below 150 percent of the federal poverty level who also meet an asset test.

About 36 percent of 2007 FFS community beneficiaries had multiple chronic conditions, about 23 percent had low income, and about 5 percent had dementia. About 50 percent of 2007 FFS community beneficiaries had at least one of these characteristics. We also examined the accuracy of the current and revised community models for beneficiaries who were not in each group to provide context for our findings.

To compare the accuracy with which the general and C-SNP new enrollee models adjust payments, we measured the accuracy of the general and C-SNP new enrollee models using the same method we used for comparing the accuracy of the current and revised community models. We used data on annualized Medicare FFS expenditures and diagnostic and demographic information for a 5 percent nationally representative, random sample of 2007 Medicare FFS new enrollees—those beneficiaries who were not enrolled in Medicare during the entire previous calendar year. We then restricted this 5 percent sample to those who, in 2007, were assigned to groups of diagnoses—called hierarchical condition categories (HCC)—that are associated with at least 1 of 14 severe or disabling chronic conditions that can be targeted by C-SNPs.[17] This methodology provided us with an estimate of the new enrollees who would have been eligible to enroll in a C-SNP in 2007.[18] Our resulting sample of C-SNP-eligible new enrollees represented about 50 percent of 2007 FFS new enrollees and about 4 percent of all FFS beneficiaries in 2007. Although C-SNP new enrollees made up less than 2 percent of all MA new enrollees and less than 0.1 percent of all MA beneficiaries in 2010, we found that about half of all 2007 FFS new enrollees would have been eligible to enroll in a C-SNP. We compared the accuracy of the general and C-SNP new enrollee models for these new enrollees (1) overall, (2) by condition, and (3) by the number of conditions.

We assessed the reliability of the Medicare data we analyzed for this report by reviewing relevant documentation, performing data checks to

---

[17] We excluded new enrollees with ESRD—1 of the 15 severe or disabling chronic conditions—from our analyses for this report because CMS uses a separate risk-adjustment model to adjust payments for MA beneficiaries with this chronic condition.

[18] Currently, each C-SNP uses its own criteria to verify that a beneficiary who wishes to enroll does have at least one of the conditions targeted by the C-SNP. CMS is in the process of developing a standardized form and guidance on verifying C-SNP eligibility. CMS expects to publish these in 2012 or 2013.

ensure that the data were reasonable and consistent, comparing the data to published sources, and interviewing CMS officials knowledgeable about the MA risk-adjustment models. We determined that the data were sufficiently reliable for the purposes of our study. Our study has three limitations. First, the accuracy of actual plan payments will depend on the characteristics of beneficiaries who enroll in MA, which may be different from the characteristics of our sample of beneficiaries who were eligible but who did not enroll in MA. Second, we used the same beneficiary sample to examine the accuracy of the community models that CMS used to develop them. As a result, for community beneficiary groups defined by characteristics included in one or both of the models, our estimated expenditures will match actual expenditures exactly. More generally, our estimates of the accuracy of health care expenditure estimates from the community models will be more accurate than estimates using data for a different beneficiary sample or for beneficiary data from later years. Third, our sample of C-SNP eligible new enrollees may not be representative of all new enrollees with severe or disabling chronic conditions because we identified these beneficiaries using major medical conditions and did not analyze individual diagnoses. However, given that there is currently variation in how C-SNPs determine beneficiary eligibility, we believe our results are a reasonable estimate of the accuracy of the general and C-SNP new enrollee models for the population of C-SNP-eligible new enrollees. (See app. II for more detail on our scope and methodology.)

We conducted this performance audit from November 2009 through November 2011 in accordance with generally accepted government auditing standards. Those standards require that we plan and perform the audit to obtain sufficient, appropriate evidence to provide a reasonable basis for our findings and conclusions based on our audit objectives. We believe that the evidence obtained provides a reasonable basis for our findings and conclusions based on our audit objectives.

Background

Research has shown that CMS's method of risk adjusting payments to MA plans to reflect beneficiary health status has become more accurate over time by including more comprehensive information on beneficiaries' health status.[19] Before 2000, CMS risk adjusted MA payments based only

---

[19]See Gregory Pope et al., "Risk Adjustment of Medicare Capitation Payments Using the CMS-HCC Model," *Health Care Financing Review*, vol. 25, no. 4 (2004): 119-141.

on beneficiaries' demographic data. From 2000 to 2003, CMS risk adjusted MA payments using a model that was based on beneficiaries' demographic characteristics and primary inpatient diagnosis associated with the principal reason for an inpatient stay. In 2004, CMS began risk adjusting payments to MA plans based on beneficiaries' demographic characteristics and major medical conditions, using a set of models called the CMS-Hierarchical Condition Category (CMS-HCC) risk-adjustment models.[20] HCCs are a way of summarizing an individual's diagnoses into major medical conditions, such as vascular disease or severe head injury.[21] CMS developed and used criteria to determine which HCCs to include in the models.[22] Certain HCCs that did not meet these criteria, such as HCCs that CMS considered particularly discretionary—susceptible to variable or inappropriate coding by providers—were excluded from the models.

The revised community model included two modifications to the current community model: it incorporated a revised set of HCCs and was calibrated with more recent data. To revise the HCCs, CMS worked with a panel of clinical experts to regroup diagnoses into HCCs, and it also reassessed which HCCs to include. This regrouping and reassessment increased the number of HCCs in the model from 70 in the current community model to 87 in the revised community model.[23] Some of the new HCCs in the revised model were previously excluded because they were considered particularly discretionary. Two examples are dementia

---

[20] CMS's use of the CMS-HCC models to adjust MA payments was phased in from 2004 to 2006. Payments to MA plans in 2007 were adjusted solely by the CMS-HCC models. These models include the community and the general new enrollee models.

[21] HCCs collapse the over 14,000 diagnosis codes into 189 clinically meaningful condition categories, some of which are additionally grouped into hierarchies of increasing severity. If a beneficiary's diagnoses correspond to more than one HCC in a hierarchy, the beneficiary is assigned only the most severe HCC in the hierarchy.

[22] For example, HCCs in the models were included in part because they increased the accuracy with which the models estimated health care expenditures. The criteria CMS used to determine which HCCs to include in the models are described in Gregory Pope et al., *Evaluation of the CMS-HCC Risk Adjustment Model Final Report* (Research Triangle Park: RTI International, March 2011).

[23] A complete list of the HCCs included in the current and revised community models is in attachment V, table 4, of CMS's "Advance Notice of Methodological Changes for Calendar Year 2011 for Medicare Advantage Capitation Rates, Part C and Part D Payment Policies and 2011 Call Letter" (Feb. 19, 2010), available at http://www.cms.gov/MedicareAdvtgSpecRateStats/AD/list.asp.

with and without complications. At the time CMS was determining which HCCs to include in the revised community model, CMS believed that benefits in improved accuracy of payment adjustments from including HCCs for dementia in the revised model outweighed the risks of introducing HCCs for which coding could be discretionary or subject to coding variation. CMS officials intended to mitigate this risk by closely monitoring the coding of dementia by comparing plans' coding of dementia with benchmarks previously established by CMS.

In March 2011, CMS published an evaluation of the CMS-HCC risk-adjustment models, as required by the 2010 Patient Protection and Affordable Care Act, which presented results on the extent to which the current and revised community models accurately estimated average actual expenditures for selected beneficiary groups.[24] The evaluation found that compared with the current community model, the revised community model, on average, was better at estimating health care expenditures for all FFS community beneficiaries.[25] The evaluation also examined the extent to which the revised community model improved accuracy for certain beneficiary groups. In particular, the evaluation found that the revised community model generally produced small changes in accuracy for beneficiaries with multiple chronic conditions, with the greatest increase in accuracy occurring for beneficiaries with 10 or more HCCs. For beneficiaries with dementia, the evaluation indicated that the revised community model—which, unlike the current community model, included two HCCs for dementia—estimated expenditures more accurately. CMS did not evaluate the performance of the revised community model for beneficiaries who received the Part D LIS and were

---

[24]The evaluation of the models is in Gregory Pope et al. *Evaluation of the CMS-HCC Risk Adjustment Model Final Report*. The current community model that CMS evaluated was based on data for 2004 and 2005, and the revised model was based on data for 2006 and 2007.

[25]The R-squared statistic is a commonly used statistic that measures the extent to which the model can explain variation in the value of its dependent variable (which is beneficiary health care expenditures in this evaluation) among individual beneficiaries. The R-squared statistic was approximately 15 percent greater in the revised community model (R-squared of 0.125) than the current community model (R-squared of 0.109). In other words, the demographic characteristics and HCCs included in the revised community model along with the more recent calibration explained about 13 percent of the total variation in estimated expenditures, while the inputs included in current community model explained about 11 percent.

not dually eligible for Medicare and Medicaid nor did it evaluate the performance of the C-SNP new enrollee model.

In April 2011, revised coding guidelines for Alzheimer's disease dementia were issued, which raised new concerns for CMS that diagnosing Alzheimer's disease dementia may be more discretionary. The revised guidelines, developed under the leadership of the National Institutes of Health and the Alzheimer's Association, expand the definition of dementia caused by Alzheimer's disease to include mild cognitive impairment and allow clincians to diagnose patients with this pre-Alzheimer's disease impairment.[26] According to CMS officials, the revised coding guidelines for Alzheimer's disease dementia increase the risk of including HCCs for dementia in the revised model because they may lead to coding variation or gaming. CMS plans to reassess whether to include HCCs for dementia in the revised model and may decide to include dementia for certain applications of the model and not others.

Effect of Revised Community Model on Payment Accuracy Varied for High-Risk Groups Studied

In our comparison of the current and revised community models, the revised community model slightly reduced the accuracy of MA payment adjustments for beneficiaries with multiple chronic conditions—one of three high-risk groups in our study. The revised community model also slightly reduced accuracy for beneficiaries with a single or no chronic conditions. Specifically, the revised community model reduced the accuracy for beneficiaries with at least two chronic conditions by $164, which was about 1 percent of average actual expenditures. Even with the reduced accuracy, for these beneficiaries the revised community model estimates, on average, were within $169 of actual expenditures, while the current community model estimates were within $5. For beneficiaries with a single or no chronic conditions, the revised community model reduced accuracy by $94, or 2 percent of average actual expenditures.

---

[26]The revised guidelines issued in April 2011 also expand the definition of Alzheimer's disease dementia to include the preclinical stage of dementia caused by Alzheimer's disease, but this stage may be used only in research settings and not by clinicians treating patients. For more information on the revised guidelines, see National Institute on Aging, *Alzheimer's Diagnostic Guidelines Updated for the First Time in Decades* (Apr. 29, 2011) accessed September 13, 2011, http://www.nia.nih.gov/Alzheimers/ResearchInformation/NewsReleases/PR20110419guidelines.htm.

While the revised community model reduced the accuracy of MA payment adjustments for beneficiaries with multiple chronic conditions as a whole, this model improved the accuracy for the 4 percent of community FFS beneficiaries with six or more chronic conditions by $727 or 2 percent of average actual expenditures. However, the revised community model still underestimated expenditures for this group by $608, about 2 percent of average actual expenditures. (See fig. 1.)

Figure 1: Accuracy of Current and Revised Community Models' Estimated Health Care Expenditures for Beneficiaries, by Number of Chronic Conditions, 2007

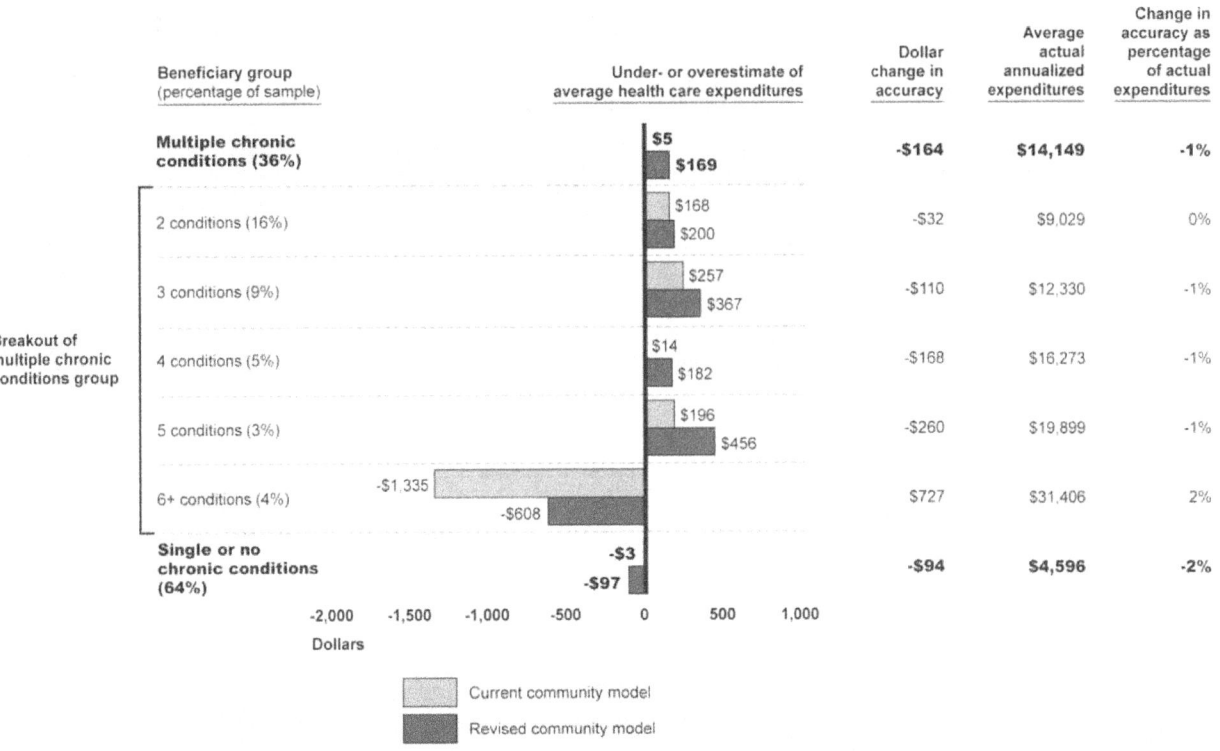

Source: GAO analysis of actual and estimated health care expenditures for a 5 percent sample of 2007 Medicare fee-for-service community beneficiaries.

Notes: The accuracy of the average estimated health expenditures for a particular group of beneficiaries was calculated by subtracting the average actual annualized Medicare expenditures in 2007 from the average estimated annual expenditures for 2007. The number of beneficiaries' chronic conditions was based on the number of hierarchical condition categories in the revised community model. See app. II for more detail on our scope and methodology.

For our second high-risk study group—beneficiaries with low income—as well as for beneficiaries who were not in this group, the revised community model produced MA payment adjustments of a similar magnitude to those produced by the current community model. Specifically, estimates from the revised model and current model differed by only $5 (less than 0.1 percent of average actual expenditures). Both models estimated expenditures for this group of low-income beneficiaries that were within $80 of actual expenditures. Within the low-income group, estimates from the revised and current community models were similar for beneficiaries who received the Part D LIS but were not dually eligible for Medicare and Medicaid, with the revised community model slightly reducing accuracy by $28, or less than 0.5 percent of average actual expenditures. Both the current and revised community models underestimated expenditures for these beneficiaries by about $450 ($435 and $463, respectively). The estimates were substantially more accurate for beneficiaries who were dual-eligibles. This greater accuracy for dual-eligibles relative to beneficiaries who received the Part D LIS but were not dually eligible reflects the design of the models: that both the current and revised community models account for whether a beneficiary is dually eligible and neither model accounts for whether a beneficiary received the Part D LIS.[27] (See fig. 2.)

---

[27] CMS considered adding a variable in the community model for LIS beneficiaries who were not dually eligible but decided not to include it. In its analysis of this variable, CMS found that the variable had a low value and did not significantly add to the model's ability to accurately estimate expenditures for these beneficiaries.

Figure 2: Accuracy of Current and Revised Community Models' Estimated Health Care Expenditures for Beneficiaries, by Income Status, 2007

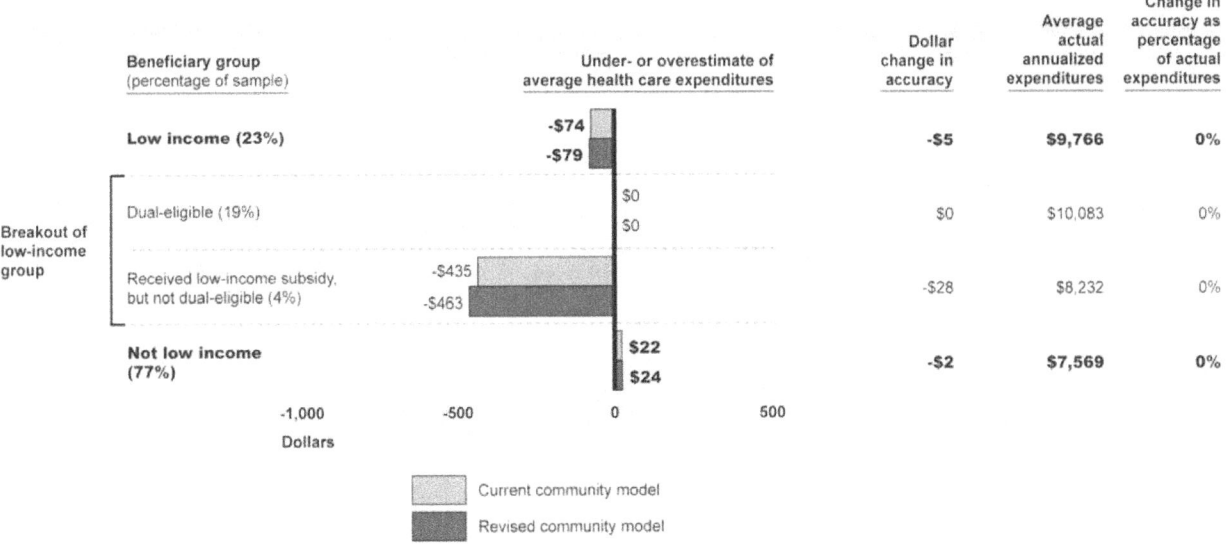

Source: GAO analysis of actual and estimated health care expenditures for a 5 percent sample of 2007 Medicare fee-for-service community beneficiaries.

Notes: The accuracy of the average estimated health expenditures for a particular group of beneficiaries was calculated by subtracting the average actual annualized Medicare expenditures in 2007 from the average estimated annual expenditures for 2007. The estimated expenditures from both the current and revised community models match actual expenditures exactly for dual-eligibles because we used the same beneficiary sample as the Centers for Medicare & Medicaid Services used to develop the model and both models account for whether a beneficiary is dually eligible for both Medicare and Medicaid. Beneficiaries who received the low-income subsidy include those with annual incomes below 150 percent of the federal poverty level who also meet an asset test. See app. II for more detail on our scope and methodology.

The revised community model produced a substantial improvement in the accuracy of health care expenditure estimates, and therefore MA payment adjustments, for the approximately 5 percent of beneficiaries diagnosed with dementia. Specifically, the revised community model improved the accuracy of estimated health care expenditures for beneficiaries with dementia by $2,674, or about 16 percent of average actual expenditures. Estimates from the revised model matched actual expenditures exactly for beneficiaries with dementia, reflecting the inclusion in the model of two new HCCs for dementia (dementia with complications and dementia without complications). The magnitude of the improvement in accuracy was greater for beneficiaries diagnosed with dementia with complications and less for beneficiaries diagnosed with dementia without complications. For the 95 percent of FFS community beneficiaries without dementia, the revised community model improved accuracy by $129, or about 2 percent of average actual expenditures. (See fig. 3.)

Figure 3: Accuracy of Current and Revised Community Models' Estimated Health Care Expenditures for Beneficiaries, by Dementia Diagnosis, 2007

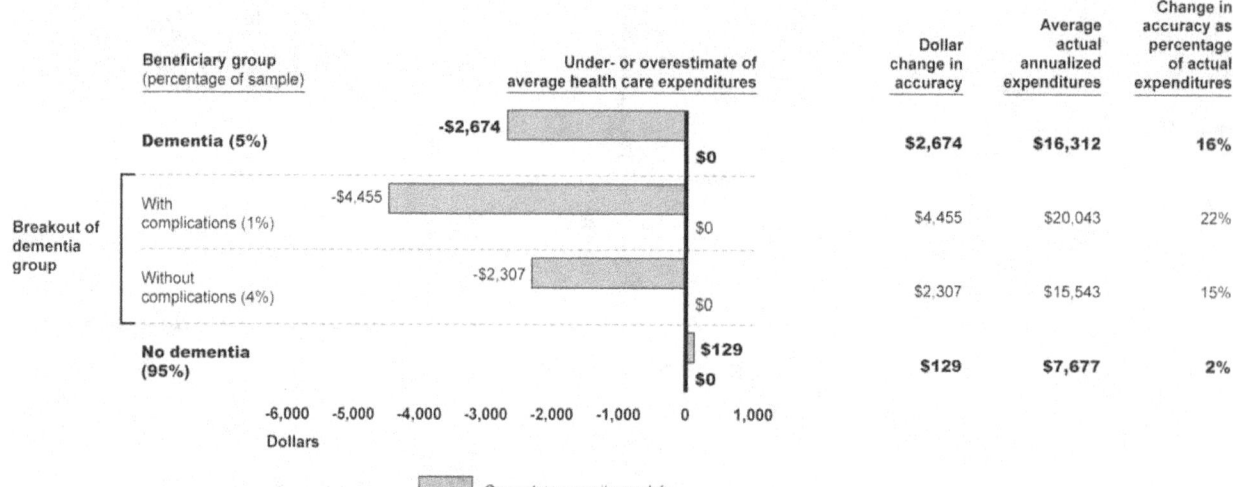

Beneficiary group (percentage of sample)	Under- or overestimate of average health care expenditures	Dollar change in accuracy	Average actual annualized expenditures	Change in accuracy as percentage of actual expenditures
Dementia (5%)	-$2,674 / $0	$2,674	$16,312	16%
Breakout of dementia group — With complications (1%)	-$4,455 / $0	$4,455	$20,043	22%
Breakout of dementia group — Without complications (4%)	-$2,307 / $0	$2,307	$15,543	15%
No dementia (95%)	$129 / $0	$129	$7,677	2%

■ Current community model
■ Revised community model

Source: GAO analysis of actual and estimated health care expenditures for a 5 percent sample of 2007 Medicare fee-for-service community beneficiaries.

Notes: The accuracy of the average estimated health expenditures for a particular group of beneficiaries was calculated by subtracting the average actual annualized Medicare expenditures in 2007 from the average estimated annual expenditures for 2007. The estimated expenditures from the revised community model match actual expenditures exactly for beneficiaries diagnosed with either of the two hierarchical condition categories (HCC) associated with dementia because we used the same beneficiary sample as the Centers for Medicare & Medicaid Services used to develop the model and we identified these beneficiaries using HCCs included in the revised community model. See app. II for more detail on our scope and methodology.

C-SNP New Enrollee Model Substantially Improved Accuracy of MA Payment Adjustments, but Considerable Inaccuracy Remains for Certain Groups

Compared with the general new enrollee model, the C-SNP new enrollee model substantially improved the accuracy of estimated health care expenditures, and therefore of MA payment adjustments, for C-SNP-eligible new enrollees but still underestimated expenditures for certain groups by considerable amounts.[28] Specifically, the C-SNP new enrollee model underestimated expenditures for C-SNP-eligible new enrollees by $1,461, while the general new enrollee model underestimated expenditures for this group by $3,914—an improvement in accuracy of $2,453, or about 25 percent of average actual expenditures. The amount by which accuracy improved was similar across 14 severe or disabling chronic conditions: $2,402 to $2,723 (a range which represented 7 to 24 percent of average actual expenditures). This result reflects the design of the C-SNP new enrollee model, which increases the expenditure estimates from the general new enrollee model by an amount that does not depend on beneficiaries' medical conditions. Despite the improved accuracy both on average and for each of the 14 conditions, the C-SNP new enrollee model still underestimated expenditures for beneficiaries who had certain conditions, such as end-stage liver disease or stroke, by more than $15,000. (See fig. 4.)

---

[28]Because CMS only uses the C-SNP new enrollee model to adjust payments for new enrollees who enroll in a C-SNP, the magnitude of the payment adjustment for new enrollees who are eligible for a C-SNP but enroll in a general MA plan will be smaller than the adjustments for C-SNP new enrollees.

Figure 4: Accuracy of General and Chronic Condition Special Needs Plan (C-SNP) New Enrollee Models' Estimated Health Care Expenditures for New Enrollees, by Severe or Disabling Chronic Condition, 2007

Beneficiary group (percentage of sample)	Under- or overestimate of average health care expenditures (General / C-SNP)	Dollar change in accuracy	Average actual annualized expenditures[b]	Change in accuracy as percentage of actual expenditures
At least one condition (100%)	-$3,914 / -$1,461	$2,453	$9,951	25%
Chronic alcohol and other drug dependence (4%)	-$16,972 / -$14,299	$2,673	$23,932	11%
Autoimmune disorders (8%)	-$5,257 / -$2,831	$2,426	$11,393	21%
Cancer[a] (18%)	-$11,341 / -$8,939	$2,402	$16,986	14%
Cardiovascular disorders (29%)	-$12,033 / -$9,582	$2,451	$18,244	13%
Chronic heart failure (13%)	-$18,351 / -$15,843	$2,508	$25,070	10%
Dementia (4%)	-$18,119 / -15,670	$2,449	$25,700	10%
Diabetes mellitus (44%)	-$4,269 / -$1,816	$2,453	$10,408	24%
End-stage liver disease (1%)	-$31,673 / -$29,027	$2,646	-$38,631	7%
Severe hematological disorders (20%)	-$14,804 / -$12,351	$2,453	$21,114	12%
Human Immunodeficiency Virus/Acquired Immodeficiency Syndrome (1%)	-$7,055 / -$4,332	$2,723	$14,000	19%
Chronic lung disorders (30%)	-$10,903 / -$8,415	$2,488	$17,412	14%
Chronic and disabling mental health conditions (14%)	-$5,743 / -$3,187	$2,556	$12,580	20%
Neurologic disorders (15%)	-$12,532 / -$10,001	$2,531	$19,172	13%
Stroke (6%)	-$19,380 / -$16,862	$2,518	$26,429	10%

Breakout of at least one condition group

■ General new enrollee model
■ C-SNP new enrollee model

Source: GAO analysis of actual and estimated health care expenditures for a 5 percent sample of 2007 Medicare fee-for-service new enrollees (beneficiaries who were not enrolled in Medicare during the entire previous calendar year).

Notes: Our sample was limited to the new enrollees who, in 2007, were assigned to hierarchical condition categories associated with at least 1 of 14 severe or disabling chronic conditions that can be targeted by C-SNPs. C-SNPs are a type of Medicare Advantage plan that is allowed to enroll only beneficiaries with certain severe or disabling chronic conditions. We excluded new enrollees with end-stage renal disease because their payments are adjusted with a separate model. The accuracy of the average estimated health expenditures for a particular group of new enrollees was calculated by subtracting the average actual annualized Medicare expenditures in 2007 from the average estimated annual expenditures for 2007. See app. II for more detail on our scope and methodology.

[a]Cancer group excludes precancer conditions and in situ status.

[b]The average actual annualized expenditures for new enrollees with at least 1 of the 14 conditions ($9,951) is less than the average actual annualized expenditures for the 14 chronic conditions individually because new enrollees with multiple conditions, especially those with 3 or more conditions who typically have high average actual annualized expenditures, are included in results for each condition (but only included once in the "at least one condition" group) and therefore make up a larger percentage of each of the 14 condition groups individually than they do for the "at least one condition" group.

Although the accuracy of MA payment adjustments with the C-SNP new enrollee model improved, both on average and by condition, the results varied depending on the number of severe or disabling conditions the new enrollees had. The C-SNP new enrollee model reduced the accuracy of expenditure estimates for the lowest-cost group of C-SNP-eligible new enrollees—those who were diagnosed with only 1 of the 14 severe or disabling chronic conditions. Specifically, the overestimate of health care expenditures for this group increased from $1,739 with the general new enrollee model to $4,160 with the C-SNP new enrollee model—a reduction in accuracy of $2,421, or about 62 percent of average actual expenditures. On the other hand, the C-SNP new enrollee model improved the accuracy of estimated health care expenditures of C-SNP eligible new enrollees with 4 or more severe or disabling conditions by $2,521, or about 8 percent of actual average expenditures. However, the C-SNP new enrollee model still underestimated expenditures for this group by over $20,000. (See fig. 5.)

Figure 5: Accuracy of General and Chronic Condition Special Needs Plan (C-SNP) New Enrollee Models' Estimated Health Care Expenditures for New Enrollees, by Number of Severe or Disabling Chronic Conditions, 2007

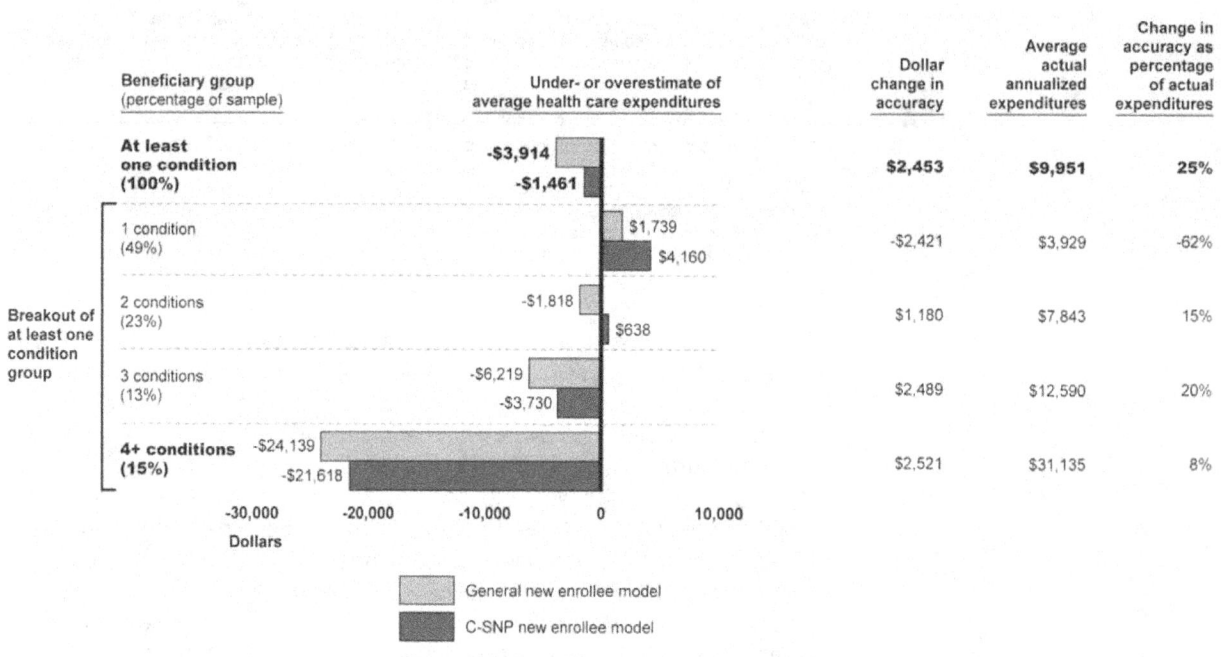

Notes: Our sample was limited to the new enrollees who, in 2007, were assigned to hierarchical condition categories associated with at least 1 of 14 severe or disabling chronic conditions that can be targeted by C-SNPs. C-SNPs are a type of Medicare Advantage plan that is allowed to enroll only beneficiaries with certain severe or disabling chronic conditions. We excluded new enrollees with end-stage renal disease because their payments are adjusted with a separate model. The accuracy of the average estimated health expenditures for a particular group of new enrollees was calculated by subtracting the average actual annualized Medicare expenditures in 2007 from the average estimated annual expenditures for 2007. See app. II for more detail on our scope and methodology.

Concluding Observations

Accurately adjusting payments to MA plans is important to help ensure that these plans have the same financial incentive to enroll and care for beneficiaries regardless of their health status or the resources they are expected to consume. Our analysis showed that compared with the current community model, the effect of CMS's revised community model on payment accuracy varied for the high-risk groups we studied. Specifically, we found that the revised model resulted in slight reductions in accuracy, on average, for beneficiaries diagnosed with multiple chronic conditions, similar levels of accuracy for beneficiaries with low income, and a substantial improvement in accuracy for beneficiaries with dementia. Recent revisions to the coding guidelines for Alzheimer's disease dementia increased CMS's concerns that there may be more coding variation or gaming for dementia. Whether CMS decides to implement the revised community model that includes HCCs for dementia will depend on CMS's assessment of the advantage of more accurate payment adjustment for beneficiaries with dementia compared with the disadvantage of a potential increase in the discretionary coding of dementia. In addition, our analysis showed that compared with the general new enrollee model, the C-SNP new enrollee model substantially improved the accuracy of payment adjustments for new enrollees diagnosed with severe or disabling conditions, on average. However, the model still considerably underestimated expenditures for new enrollees diagnosed with four or more severe or disabling conditions, which could place plans that disproportionately enroll these beneficiaries at a relative financial disadvantage.

Agency Comments and Our Evaluation

CMS provided written comments on a draft of this report, which are reprinted in appendix III.

In its comments, CMS suggested that the report include an assessment of the overall accuracy of the current risk adjustment model. While we agree that an overall assessment of the model's accuracy would be useful, such an analysis was not within the scope of our work and would have required additional data.

CMS stated that the report places considerable focus on the C-SNP new enrollee model even though there were fewer than 10,000 C-SNP new enrollees in 2010. One of the study's main objectives was to compare the accuracy of CMS' C-SNP model for new enrollees with the general new enrollee model. Moreover, we note that 50 percent of the 2007 FFS new enrollee population was eligible to enroll in a C-SNP.

In addition, CMS suggested that the report should include an evaluation of whether the differences in the current and revised risk adjustment models are statistically significant or meaningful. We did not test for statistical differences because we used a large sample, and note that CMS also did not test for statistical differences in its evaluation of the risk adjustment model.[29] We do report dollar differences in the estimates to allow readers to make their own judgments as to whether these differences are large enough to be meaningful.

Finally, CMS commented that the community risk-adjustment models do not include a coefficient for beneficiaries who received the Part D LIS but were not dually eligible because CMS found that such a coefficient was small and not statistically significant. We have included a footnote to that effect in the report.

As agreed with your offices, unless you publicly announce the contents of this report earlier, we plan no further distribution until 30 days from the report date. At that time, we will send copies to the Secretary of HHS, interested congressional committees, and others. In addition, the report will be available at no charge on the GAO website at http://www.gao.gov. If you or your staff have any questions about this report, please contact me at (202) 512-7114 or cosgrovej@gao.gov. Contact points for our Offices of Congressional Relations and Public Affairs may be found on the last page of this report. GAO staff who made major contributions to this report are listed in appendix IV.

James C. Cosgrove
Director, Health Care

---

[29]See Gregory Pope et al., *Evaluation of the CMS-HCC Risk Adjustment Model Final Report* (Research Triangle Park: RTI International, March 2011).

List of Requesters

The Honorable Henry A. Waxman
Ranking Member
Committee on Energy and Commerce
House of Representatives

The Honorable Frank Pallone, Jr.
Ranking Member
Subcommittee on Health
Committee on Energy and Commerce
House of Representatives

The Honorable Pete Stark
Ranking Member
Subcommittee on Health
Committee on Ways and Means
House of Representatives

The Honorable John D. Dingell
The Honorable Charles B. Rangel
House of Representatives

Appendix I: Additional Potential Changes to the Medicare Advantage Risk-Adjustment Models

The Centers for Medicare & Medicaid Services (CMS) has been conducting ongoing research on the Medicare Advantage (MA) risk-adjustment models to improve the models' accuracy in estimating expenditures for beneficiary groups. A major focus of CMS's research is modifying the models to ensure that they accurately estimate expenditures for high-cost beneficiaries and therefore encourage high-quality care for them. The modifications that CMS proposed in 2010—to revise the diagnoses included in the community model and to introduce the chronic condition special needs plan new enrollee model—are results of this ongoing research.

The following tables present some of these potential changes to the MA risk-adjustment models that CMS considered and describe CMS's rationale for not implementing them. The tables group the potential changes into three categories: table 1 presents the changes that involved adding new variables to the models, table 2 describes new information sources that CMS considered using, and table 3 presents the changes that involved changing the models' structure.

Appendix I: Additional Potential Changes to the Medicare Advantage Risk-Adjustment Models

Table 1: Potential Changes to the Medicare Advantage (MA) Risk-Adjustment Models: Adding Variables to the Models

Model change	Description of change and rationale for consideration	Centers for Medicare & Medicaid Services' (CMS) rationale for not implementing
Functional status (or frailty) adjustment	To adjust payments for the frail elderly, CMS considered revising the model by adding variables that would measure functional status based on the number of activities of daily living (ADL), such as bathing or eating, that each MA beneficiary had difficulty performing.[a,b] According to one study, the community model, on average, underestimated expenditures for beneficiaries with ADL limitations.[c]	CMS does not have access to individual-level data on ADLs for all beneficiaries.
Comorbidity count adjustment	To adjust payments for beneficiaries with multiple chronic conditions, CMS analyzed including a variable to the community model that would indicate the total number of chronic conditions for each beneficiary. This variable could account for the possibility that because of interactions among chronic conditions, total expenditures for beneficiaries with multiple chronic conditions are, on average, greater than the sum of estimated expenditures associated with each condition separately.[d]	CMS found that adding a variable indicating the number of comorbid conditions for each beneficiary did not substantially improve the models' ability to estimate expenditures, except for beneficiaries with seven or more conditions. Additionally, the current and revised community models already adjust for the additional effect of interactions between certain comorbid conditions on total expenditures by including six disease interaction terms (such as the interaction between diabetes and congestive heart failure). CMS has been conducting ongoing research to assess which additional interaction terms may be added to the CMS-Hierarchical Condition Category risk-adjustment models to improve the models' predictive accuracy.
Mortality adjustment	CMS considered adjusting MA payments for mortality to help account for the increased expenditures associated with end-of-life care. One study found that average annual Medicare expenditures for beneficiaries who died were six times greater than those for beneficiaries who survived.[e]	CMS did not implement a mortality adjustment because of concerns that paying MA plans more for beneficiaries who died would introduce an inappropriate financial incentive.

Sources: Interviews with CMS officials and contractors and Gregory Pope, John Kautter, Melvin Ingber, Sara Freeman, Rishi Sekar, and Cordon Newhart, *Evaluation of the CMS-HCC Risk Adjustment Model*, Final report (March 2011).

[a]For more information about the functional status adjustment, see John Kautter and Gregory Pope, "CMS Frailty Adjustment Model," *Health Care Financing Review*, vol. 26 no. 2 (2004-2005): 1-19, and Gregory Pope, John Kautter, Melvin Ingber, Sara Freeman, Rishi Sekar, and Cordon Newhart, *Evaluation of the CMS-HCC Risk Adjustment Model*, Final report.

[b]Using data from the Medicare Health Outcomes Survey, which is based on a sample of Medicare beneficiaries, CMS currently applies a contract-level frailty adjustment for beneficiaries age 55 or older who are enrolled in Program of All-Inclusive Care for the Elderly (PACE) organizations. PACE organizations are managed care plans outside of MA that provide Medicare and Medicaid services as well as some social services, such as nutritional counseling. In 2012, CMS will begin using the frailty adjustment for fully integrated dual-eligible special needs plans, which provide Medicare and Medicaid benefits and contract with state Medicaid agencies for services such as long-term care for plans that have similar average levels of frailty as PACE organizations.

[c]See Katia Noyes, Hangsheng Liu, and Helena Temkin-Greener, "Medicare Capitation Model, Functional Status, and Multiple Comorbidities: Model Accuracy," *The American Journal of Managed Care*, vol. 14, no. 10 (2008): 679-690.

[d]See Jennifer Wolff, Barbara Starfield, and Gerard Anderson, "Prevalence, Expenditures, and Complications of Multiple Chronic Conditions in the Elderly," *Archives of Internal Medicine*, vol. 162 (2002): 2269-2276, and Bianca Frogner, Gerard Anderson, Robb Cohen, and Chad Abrams, "Incorporating New Research Into Medicare Risk Adjustment," *Medical Care*, vol. 49, no. 3 (2011): 295-300.

Appendix I: Additional Potential Changes to
the Medicare Advantage Risk-Adjustment
Models

[e]See Christopher Hogan, June Lunney, Jon Gabel, and Joanne Lynn, "Medicare Beneficiaries' Costs of Care in the Last Year of Life," *Health Affairs*, vol. 20, no. 4, (2001): 188–195.

Table 2: Potential Changes to the Medicare Advantage (MA) Risk-Adjustment Models: Adding New Information Sources

Model change	Description of change and rationale for consideration	Centers for Medicare & Medicaid Services' (CMS) rationale for not implementing
Two years of data to identify chronic conditions	CMS assessed the implications of revising the model to include data for 2 years before the payment year to potentially adjust MA payments for some chronic conditions that were diagnosed 2 years—but not 1 year—before the payment year. Once an MA beneficiary is diagnosed with a chronic condition that is included in the CMS-Hierarchical Condition Category risk-adjustment models, the MA plan will continue to be at risk for all expenditures for this beneficiary for this condition during any subsequent years of MA enrollment because chronic conditions persist over time. However, for any subsequent year(s) during which an MA provider does not diagnose the beneficiary with that condition, MA payments will not be adjusted for that condition during the following (payment) year. One study found that five chronic diseases were diagnosed approximately 14 to 38 percent more frequently (depending on the disease) when 2 consecutive years of diagnostic data were used instead of 1 year of data.[a]	CMS assessed results from a model that used 2 years of diagnostic data to identify hierarchical condition categories (HCC) and found that it did not improve the model's accuracy in estimating expenditures. In addition, a CMS official expressed concerns about paying MA plans for HCCs that were not treated during the most recent calendar year.
Medicare Part D prescription drug data	CMS considered including Medicare Part D data—data from Medicare's prescription drug benefit program—in the risk-adjustment model to identify HCCs that were treated with prescription drugs in the year preceding the payment year but that were not diagnosed by a provider during that time. Medicare Part D data could potentially identify diagnosed chronic conditions for beneficiaries who used a prescription drug to treat a condition and did not have a physician, hospital, or nonphysician visit for that condition.	CMS found that incorporating prescription drug data in the model produced only a minimal improvement in the models' accuracy in estimating expenditures but that those modest gains were outweighed by limitations. According to CMS officials, one limitation is that the vast majority of prescription drugs are used to treat multiple conditions, and without additional information, it is not clear which condition was present. CMS also expressed concerns that using Part D data could create incentives for MA providers to prescribe drugs.
Diagnostic data on use of durable medical equipment (DME)	CMS considered including diagnostic data from DME vendors, as well as indicators of DME use, such as use of oxygen therapy and wheelchairs, to identify frail beneficiaries. According to one study, the community model, on average, underestimated expenditures for beneficiaries with activities of daily living (ADL) limitations.[b] Another study found that most noninstitutionalized beneficiaries age 65 and older who used a wheelchair had at least one ADL.[c]	CMS found that using DME data modestly improved the model's predictive accuracy but expressed concern that use of these data could promote the inappropriate use of DME.

Sources: Interviews with CMS officials and Gregory Pope, John Kautter, Melvin Ingber, Sara Freeman, Rishi Sekar, and Cordon Newhart, *Evaluation of the CMS-HCC Risk Adjustment Model*, Final report (March 2011).

[a]See Bianca Frogner, Gerard Anderson, Robb Cohen, and Chad Abrams, "Incorporating New Research Into Medicare Risk Adjustment," *Medical Care*, vol. 49, no. 3 (2011): 295-300.

[b]See Katia Noyes, Hangsheng Liu, and Helena Temkin-Greener, "Medicare Capitation Model, Functional Status, and Multiple Comorbidities: Model Accuracy," *The American Journal of Managed Care*, vol. 14, no. 10 (2008): 679-690.

Appendix I: Additional Potential Changes to the Medicare Advantage Risk-Adjustment Models

[c]See H. Stephen Kaye, Taewoon Kang, and Michelle LaPlante, "Mobility Device Use in the United States," *Disability Statistics Report*, vol. 14 (Washington, D.C.: U.S. Department of Education, National Institute on Disability and Rehabilitation Research, June 2000).

Table 3: Potential Changes to the Medicare Advantage (MA) Risk-Adjustment Models: Changing Models' Structure

Model change	Description of change and rationale for consideration	Centers for Medicare & Medicaid's Services' (CMS) rationale for not implementing
Separate model for beneficiaries with no hierarchical condition categories (HCC)	CMS considered using a separate model for beneficiaries with no HCCs.[a] It is difficult for linear regression models, such as the CMS-Hierarchical Condition Categories (CMS-HCC) risk-adjustment models, to accurately predict expenditures for beneficiaries with zero expenditures, an outcome present for many beneficiaries with no HCCs. To account for beneficiaries who have zero expenditures, one approach is to estimate a nonlinear expenditure model for beneficiaries with zero Medicare expenditures and another model for beneficiaries with positive Medicare expenditures.[b]	CMS found that using separate models depending on whether beneficiaries had been diagnosed with an HCC resulted in larger values for some of the demographic variables in the model for beneficiaries with no HCCs. In these cases, some MA plans could have an incentive to refrain from reporting an HCC to receive a higher payment.
Use concurrent models	CMS assessed the advantages and disadvantages of concurrent risk-adjustment models. One advantage of concurrent models according to one study is that they estimate expenditures more accurately compared with prospective models, such as the CMS-HCC risk-adjustment models.[c] Concurrent risk-adjustment models use payment year diagnoses to estimate payment year expenditures. Prospective models use diagnoses from the calendar year before the payment year to estimate expenditures.	According to CMS officials, concurrent models give more weight to acute conditions than prospective models, and risk-adjustment models should primarily adjust for chronic conditions and systemic risks because they can be managed better than acute conditions. Concurrent models do not estimate expenditures for chronic conditions more accurately than those for prospective models, and concurrent models would delay payments to MA plans.
Nonlinear functional form	CMS considered using a nonlinear functional form for the MA risk-adjustment model that would account for expenditures associated with additional combinations of comorbid conditions because it could potentially improve expenditure estimates for beneficiaries with multiple chronic conditions. One study found that the MA risk-adjustment model underestimates expenditures, on average, for some groups of beneficiaries who have multiple chronic conditions.[d]	CMS found that the nonlinear model it tested did not, in general, improve the predictive accuracy of expenditure estimates. In addition, CMS concluded that nonlinear models were more difficult to explain and estimate.

Sources: Interviews with CMS officials and Gregory Pope, John Kautter, Melvin Ingber, Sara Freeman, Rishi Sekar, and Cordon Newhart, *Evaluation of the CMS-HCC Risk Adjustment Model*, Final report (March 2011).

[a]HCCs are a way of summarizing an individual's diagnoses into major medical conditions, such as vascular disease or severe head injury.

[b]For more information, see Melinda Buntin and Alan Zaslavsky, "Too Much Ado About Two-Part Models and Transformation? Comparing Methods of Modeling Medicare Expenditures," *Journal of Health Economics*, vol. 23 (2004): 525-542.

[c]For more information, see R. Adams Dudley, Carol Medlin, Lisa Hammann, Miriam Cisternas, Richard Brand, Deborah Renne, and Harold Luft, "The Best of Both Worlds? Potential of Hybrid Prospective/Concurrent Risk Adjustment," *Medical Care*, vol. 41, no. 1 (2003): 56-60.

[d]See Katia Noyes, Hangsheng Liu, and Helena Temkin-Greener, "Medicare Capitation Model, Functional Status, and Multiple Comorbidities: Model Accuracy," *The American Journal of Managed Care*, vol. 14, no. 10 (2008): 679-690.

Appendix II: Scope and Methodology

This appendix describes the scope and methodology we used to address our two objectives: to compare (1) the accuracy with which the current and revised community models adjust Medicare Advantage (MA) payments to account for differences in beneficiaries' expected health care expenditures and (2) the accuracy with which the general and chronic condition special needs plan (C-SNP)[1] new enrollee models adjust MA payments to account for differences in beneficiaries' expected health care expenditures.

Comparing the Accuracy of Current and Revised Community Models

To compare the accuracy with which the current and revised community models would adjust MA payments, we computed the amount by which health care expenditure estimates from the current and revised community models were above or below actual expenditures. We calculated the accuracy of the average estimated health expenditures for a particular group of beneficiaries by subtracting the group's average actual annualized Medicare expenditures in 2007 from the group's average estimated expenditures for 2007.[2] We considered the revised community model an improvement in accuracy of MA payment adjustments if the magnitude of the over- or underestimate of health care expenditures from the revised community model was smaller than the over- or underestimate from the current community model.

For our analysis, we used versions of the current and revised community models that were calibrated with the same data (Medicare fee-for-service (FFS) data for 2006 and 2007) and therefore differed only in the

---

[1] C-SNPs are plans that only enroll beneficiaries with at least 1 of 15 severe or disabling chronic conditions: chronic alcohol and other drug dependence, autoimmune disorders, cancer (excluding precancer conditions or in situ status), cardiovascular disorders, chronic heart failure, dementia, diabetes mellitus, end-stage liver disease, end-stage renal disease (ESRD), severe hematological disorders, Human Immunodeficiency Virus/Acquired Immunodeficiency Syndrome, chronic lung disorders, chronic and disabling mental health conditions, neurologic disorders, and stroke. The 15 conditions were defined by a panel of clinical advisors convened by the Centers for Medicare & Medicaid Services.

[2] Each beneficiary's contribution to the group's average estimated or actual expenditures was weighted by the number of months each beneficiary met the definition of a community beneficiary.

Appendix II: Scope and Methodology

hierarchical condition categories (HCC) that were included in the models.[3] Because we compared versions of the current and revised community models calibrated on the same data, our results reflect only the impact of the clinical revisions to the HCCs and not the recalibration that the Centers for Medicare & Medicaid Services (CMS) performs on a periodic basis.[4]

Our study population consisted of a 5 percent nationally representative, random sample of 2007 Medicare FFS community beneficiaries—FFS beneficiaries who, if they had enrolled in an MA plan, would have had their 2007 payments adjusted by the community model.[5] We used Medicare FFS data because health care expenditure data were not available for MA beneficiaries,[6] and we used data from 2007 because this was the most recent version of these data available at the time we began our study. For each beneficiary, we obtained the inputs to the community model (selected demographic characteristics and medical diagnoses from the previous year),[7] actual annualized 2007 FFS expenditures, and the portion of the year for which plan payments for the beneficiary would have

---

[3]HCCs group an individual's diagnoses into major medical conditions, such as vascular disease or severe head injury. HCCs collapse the over 14,000 diagnosis codes into 189 clinically meaningful condition categories, some of which are additionally grouped into hierarchies of increasing severity. If a beneficiary's diagnoses correspond to more than one HCC in a hierarchy, the beneficiary is assigned only the most severe HCC in the hierarchy.

[4]The revised community model was calibrated with 2006-2007 Medicare FFS data, while the model CMS used in 2009 through 2011 was calibrated with 2004-2005 data and the model CMS used in 2004 through 2008 was calibrated with 1999-2000 data.

[5]Community beneficiaries are those with a complete year of Medicare Part B enrollment during the previous calendar year who have not been diagnosed with ESRD and have not been residing in an institution, such as a nursing home, for the past 90 consecutive days or more.

[6]CMS will begin requiring MA plans to submit health care expenditure data to CMS in 2012. According to a CMS official, CMS does not plan on using these MA data to estimate the risk-adjustment model until at least 3 or 4 years of encounter data have been collected from all MA plans.

[7]Because the community model is a prospective model, expenditure estimates from one year are based on the beneficiary's characteristics in the previous year. Accordingly, for our sample of 2007 Medicare FFS community beneficiaries, we used beneficiaries' 2006 characteristics to estimate their 2007 expenditures.

Appendix II: Scope and Methodology

been adjusted using the community model.[8] We then used these inputs and the versions of the community models described above to estimate Medicare's 2007 health care expenditures on behalf of each beneficiary.

Within our 5 percent sample of community beneficiaries, we separately compared the accuracy of the current and revised community models for three high-risk beneficiary groups. We defined these three groups as follows based on their characteristics in the previous year:

- assigned to at least two of the HCCs in the revised community model,

- dually eligible for Medicare and Medicaid or received the Part D low-income subsidy,[9] and

- assigned to at least one of the two HCCs in the revised community model associated with dementia: dementia with complications and dementia without complications.

For each high-risk group, we also examined the accuracy of the current and revised community models for beneficiaries who were not in that group to provide context for our findings. For example, in addition to examining the models' accuracy for community beneficiaries with multiple chronic conditions, we also examined accuracy for beneficiaries with a single chronic condition or no chronic conditions.

Comparing the Accuracy of General and C-SNP New Enrollee Models

To compare the accuracy with which the general and C-SNP new enrollee models adjust payments for C-SNP-eligible new enrollees, we measured the accuracy of the general and C-SNP new enrollee models using the same method we used for comparing the accuracy of the current and revised community models. Similar to our community model

---

[8] To be consistent with the types of expenditures that CMS uses to calibrate the current and revised community models, we excluded expenditures for months when the beneficiary was enrolled in an MA plan, receiving hospice care, residing in a nursing home for at least the previous 90 days, or entitled to Medicare because of having ESRD. These excluded expenditures are either adjusted for by a different risk-adjustment model or correspond to hospice services for which MA plans do not pay.

[9] The Part D low-income subsidy program provides financial assistance to beneficiaries with limited income and assets. Eligible beneficiaries include those with annual incomes below 150 percent of the federal poverty level who also meet an asset test. To identify these beneficiaries, we used data from Acumen, a CMS contractor.

Appendix II: Scope and Methodology

analysis, we used versions of the general and C-SNP new enrollee models that were derived using Medicare FFS data for 2006 and 2007.[10] To identify our study population, we started with a 5 percent nationally representative, random sample of 2007 Medicare FFS new enrollees—those beneficiaries who were not enrolled in Medicare Part B during the entire previous calendar year. We then restricted this sample of new enrollees to those who, in 2007, were assigned to HCCs associated with at least 1 of 14 severe or disabling chronic conditions that can be targeted by C-SNPs.[11] This methodology provided us with an estimate of the new enrollees who would have been eligible to enroll in a C-SNP in 2007.[12] We compared the accuracy of the general and C-SNP new enrollee models for these new enrollees (1) overall, (2) by condition, and (3) by number of conditions.

Data Reliability and Limitations

We assessed the reliability of the Medicare data we used for this report by reviewing relevant documentation, performing data checks, and interviewing CMS officials knowledgeable about the CMS-Hierarchical Condition Category (CMS-HCC) risk-adjustment models. We checked our data in three major ways. First, we verified that the beneficiaries in the 5 percent community and new enrollee sample files met their respective

---

[10]Because CMS had not yet calculated the C-SNP new enrollee model coefficients based on 2006-2007 data, we estimated them. To do so, we used (1) coefficients for both the general and C-SNP new enrollee models based on 2004-2005 data and (2) coefficients for the general new enrollee model, which were based on 2006-2007 data. Specifically, we calculated the percentage increase between the 2004-2005 coefficients for the general new enrollee model and the C-SNP new enrollee models and then increased the 2006-2007 general new enrollee model coefficients by this percentage.

[11]To identify these beneficiaries, we used a modified version of a list published by CMS that mapped the severe or disabling chronic conditions to the corresponding HCCs in the revised community model. The mapping published by CMS contained HCCs included in the revised community model, other HCCs not included in the model, and subsets of certain HCCs. (See Gregory Pope, John Kautter, Melvin Ingber, Sara Freeman, Rishi Sekar, and Cordon Newhart, *Evaluation of the CMS-HCC Risk Adjustment Model*, Final report (March 2011).) We adapted CMS's mapping approach for the revised community model by using complete HCCs in the place of subsets of HCCs and only using HCCs included in the revised community model. We excluded new enrollees with ESRD because their payments are adjusted with a separate model.

[12]Currently, each C-SNP uses its own criteria to verify that a beneficiary who wishes to enroll has at least one of the conditions targeted by the C-SNP. CMS is in the process of developing a standardized form and guidance on verifying C-SNP eligibility. CMS expects to publish these in 2012 or 2013.

Appendix II: Scope and Methodology

inclusion criteria. Second, we verified that we were using the CMS-HCC risk-adjustment models correctly by checking the values of the estimated expenditures and assigned HCCs for several beneficiaries. Third, for beneficiary groups in our analysis that CMS also included in its evaluation, we compared our results with those published by CMS. We determined that the data were sufficiently reliable for the purposes of our study.

Our study has three limitations. First, the accuracy of actual plan payments will depend on the characteristics of beneficiaries who enroll in MA, which may be different from the characteristics of our sample of beneficiaries who were eligible but who did not enroll in an MA plan. Second, we used the same beneficiary sample to examine the accuracy of the community models as CMS used to develop the community models. As a result, for community beneficiary groups defined by characteristics included in one or more of the models,[13] our estimated expenditures will match actual expenditures exactly. More generally, our estimates of the accuracy of health care expenditure estimates from the community models will be more accurate than estimates using data for a different beneficiary sample or for beneficiary data from later years. Third, our sample of C-SNP-eligible new enrollees may not be representative of all new enrollees with severe or disabling chronic conditions because we identified these beneficiaries using HCCs and did not analyze underlying diagnoses. However, given that there is currently variation in how C-SNPs determine beneficiary eligibility, we believe our results are a reasonable estimate of the accuracy of the general and C-SNP new enrollee models for the population of C-SNP eligible new enrollees.

We conducted this performance audit from November 2009 through November 2011 in accordance with generally accepted government auditing standards. Those standards require that we plan and perform the audit to obtain sufficient, appropriate evidence to provide a reasonable basis for our findings and conclusions based on our audit objectives. We believe that the evidence obtained provides a reasonable basis for our findings and conclusions based on our audit objectives.

---

[13]Beneficiary groups in our analysis that were defined by characteristics included in one or more of the models are beneficiaries diagnosed with dementia with or without complications—a characteristic only included in the revised community model—and beneficiaries who are eligible for both Medicare and Medicaid—a characteristic included in both the current and revised community models.

Appendix III: Comments from the Centers for Medicare & Medicaid Services

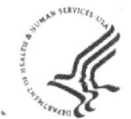

DEPARTMENT OF HEALTH & HUMAN SERVICES OFFICE OF THE SECRETARY

Assistant Secretary for Legislation
Washington, DC 20201

James Cosgrove, Director
Health Care
U.S. Government Accountability Office
441 G Street NW
Washington, DC 20548

NOV 0 3 2011

Dear Mr. Cosgrove:

Attached are comments on the U.S. Government Accountability Office's (GAO) draft report entitled, "MEDICARE ADVANTAGE: Changes Improved Accuracy of Risk Adjustment for Certain Beneficiaries" (GAO-12-52).

The Department appreciates the opportunity to review this report prior to publication.

Sincerely,

Jim R. Esquea
Assistant Secretary for Legislation

Attachment

Appendix III: Comments from the Centers for Medicare & Medicaid Services

GENERAL COMMENTS OF THE DEPARTMENT OF HEALTH AND HUMAN SERVICES (HHS) ON THE GOVERNMENT ACCOUNTABILITY OFFICE'S (GAO) DRAFT REPORT ENTITLED, "MEDICARE ADVANTAGE: CHANGES IMPROVED ACCURACY OF RISK ADJUSTMENT FOR CERTAIN BENEFICIARIES" (GAO-12-52)

The Department appreciates the opportunity to review and comment on this draft report.

The Centers for Medicare and Medicaid Services (CMS) believe that the report shows that the current risk adjustment model being used for Medicare Advantage (MA) payments is quite accurate. In particular, figure 1 shows that the predicted expenditures for the current model are within 2 percent of expenditures for 96 percent of the enrollees, and within 4 percent for individuals with six or more chronic conditions.

Accuracy of Current Model, Using Data from Figure 1 (page 14) of GAO Report

Number of Chronic Conditions	Percent of Beneficiaries	Under or Over estimate of Average Health Care Expenditures	Average Actual Annualized Expenditures	Percent Over or Under Prediction
Single or no conditions	0.64	-$3	$4,596	-0.1%
2 conditions	0.16	$168	$9,029	1.9%
3 conditions	0.09	$257	$12,330	2.1%
4 conditions	0.05	$14	$16,273	0.1%
5 conditions	0.03	$196	$19,899	1.0%
6+ conditions	0.04	-$1,335	$31,406	-4.3%

The GAO lists two objectives in the report. The first objective is to compare the risk adjustment model CMS currently uses for community-residing beneficiaries and the revised model originally proposed for use in payment year 2011. The second objective is to evaluate the C-SNP model. In addition, page 4 of the report notes that the GAO was asked "to examine how accurately the MA risk-adjustment models estimate health care expenditures, especially for high-risk beneficiary groups. As such, CMS suggests that the report include, before comparing the two versions of the model, an assessment of the accuracy of the existing risk adjustment model itself. For example, in several places within the findings, the GAO includes comparative results on the models. However, GAO does not make any statements about whether or not the existing risk model accurately predicts costs. Without the context of the overall model performance, comments comparing the accuracy of the two versions of the models may be difficult to interpret. As noted in the figure shown above, the existing model is very accurate for individuals with multiple chronic conditions.

The introduction of the report includes a considerable focus on the C-SNP new enrollee model. A small proportion of enrollees are in C-SNPs, as compared to the entire MA

Appendix III: Comments from the Centers for
Medicare & Medicaid Services

GENERAL COMMENTS OF THE DEPARTMENT OF HEALTH AND HUMAN SERVICES (HHS) ON THE GOVERNMENT ACCOUNTABILITY OFFICE'S (GAO) DRAFT REPORT ENTITLED, "MEDICARE ADVANTAGE: CHANGES IMPROVED ACCURACY OF RISK ADJUSTMENT FOR CERTAIN BENEFICIARIES" (GAO-12-52)

program, and an even smaller proportion are new enrollees. CMS provided these numbers to the GAO in July, 2011. The numbers are shown below. Less than ten thousand MA enrollees are paid with the C-SNP new enrollee model.

July 2010 C-SNP Enrollment by Beneficiary Type
Excludes ESRD and Hospice

Beneficiary Type	Number	Percent
Community	220,387	95.8%
Institutional	1,087	0.5%
New Enrollees	8,552	3.7%

July 2010 MA Enrollment by Beneficiary Type
Excludes ESRD and Hospice

Beneficiary Type	Number	Percent
Community	9,765,098	93.4%
Institutional	118,079	1.1%
New Enrollees	573,155	5.5%

The results include several findings that show one model is either more or less accurate than the other, and include dollar figures to reach this conclusion. For example, on page 13, the GAO states that "the revised community model reduced the accuracy of estimated Medicare expenditures for beneficiaries with at least 2 chronic conditions by $164, which was about 1 percent of average actual expenditures". We suggest that GAO also evaluate whether or not the differences in the models are either statistically significant, or represent meaningful differences. A difference of 1 percent, for example, is probably not meaningful or statistically significant. The GAO reports a $5 change in the under-estimation of cost as a reduction in accuracy, however, it seems that $5 is below the accuracy level of the study. In other words, CMS expects that there would be a minimum threshold set to determine if the model was more or less accurate, and $5 appears to be below what CMS would expect that threshold to be.

On page 16, the GAO compares the dual eligibles with beneficiaries who received the Part D subsidy but were not dual eligibles. CMS evaluated whether or not to include a coefficient for these the non-dual eligibles within the CMS-HCC model, and found that the model coefficient was small and not statistically significant. As a result, were the coefficient included in the model, CMS would overpay for the non-dual eligible group and underpay for the dual eligible group.

Appendix IV: GAO Contact and Staff Acknowledgments

GAO Contact	James C. Cosgrove, (202) 512-7114 or cosgrovej@gao.gov
Staff Acknowledgments	In addition to the contact named above, Christine Brudevold, Assistant Director; Alison Binkowski; William Black; Andrew Johnson; Richard Lipinski; Elizabeth Morrison; Merrile Sing; and James Walker, Jr. made key contributions to this report.

GAO's Mission	The Government Accountability Office, the audit, evaluation, and investigative arm of Congress, exists to support Congress in meeting its constitutional responsibilities and to help improve the performance and accountability of the federal government for the American people. GAO examines the use of public funds; evaluates federal programs and policies; and provides analyses, recommendations, and other assistance to help Congress make informed oversight, policy, and funding decisions. GAO's commitment to good government is reflected in its core values of accountability, integrity, and reliability.
Obtaining Copies of GAO Reports and Testimony	The fastest and easiest way to obtain copies of GAO documents at no cost is through GAO's website (www.gao.gov). Each weekday afternoon, GAO posts on its website newly released reports, testimony, and correspondence. To have GAO e-mail you a list of newly posted products, go to www.gao.gov and select "E-mail Updates."
Order by Phone	The price of each GAO publication reflects GAO's actual cost of production and distribution and depends on the number of pages in the publication and whether the publication is printed in color or black and white. Pricing and ordering information is posted on GAO's website, http://www.gao.gov/ordering.htm. Place orders by calling (202) 512-6000, toll free (866) 801-7077, or TDD (202) 512-2537. Orders may be paid for using American Express, Discover Card, MasterCard, Visa, check, or money order. Call for additional information.
Connect with GAO	Connect with GAO on Facebook, Flickr, Twitter, and YouTube. Subscribe to our RSS Feeds or E-mail Updates. Listen to our Podcasts. Visit GAO on the web at www.gao.gov.
To Report Fraud, Waste, and Abuse in Federal Programs	Contact: Website: www.gao.gov/fraudnet/fraudnet.htm E-mail: fraudnet@gao.gov Automated answering system: (800) 424-5454 or (202) 512-7470
Congressional Relations	Ralph Dawn, Managing Director, dawnr@gao.gov, (202) 512-4400 U.S. Government Accountability Office, 441 G Street NW, Room 7125 Washington, DC 20548
Public Affairs	Chuck Young, Managing Director, youngc1@gao.gov, (202) 512-4800 U.S. Government Accountability Office, 441 G Street NW, Room 7149 Washington, DC 20548

Please Print on Recycled Paper

www.ingramcontent.com/pod-product-compliance
Lightning Source LLC
Chambersburg PA
CBHW081245180526
45171CB00005B/542